Ctrl+Z Your Age

The Geek's Manual to Human Debugging

Volodymyr Rybaiev

Table of Contents

You've Got Mail: Decoding Your Body's Messages

Alright, listen up, fellow keyboard warriors! Before we dive headfirst into the matrix of human debugging, we need to talk about something crucial: **communication**. And no, I don't mean upping your Twitter game or finally responding to those LinkedIn messages from recruiters offering you a hot new gig in *checks notes* underwater basket weaving.

I'm talking about the most important communication network you'll ever hack into—your own body.

The Inbox: Understanding Your Body's Signals

You know how your email inbox has a bazillion messages, some important, some pure spam? Your body works the same way. It's constantly sending you signals, trying to tell you what's up, what's wrong, and what needs fixing. But here's the kicker: **most of us are worse at checking our bodily messages than we are at checking our emails**. And that's saying something, considering I've seen inboxes that could make a grown IT guy cry.

The Subject Line: Symptoms 101

Symptoms, my friends, are your body's subject lines. They're the quick, eye-catching summaries of what's going on under the hood. Here are a few examples:

- **Feeling like you've been hit by a truck**: *Subject: Possible flu alert!*

- **Pounding headache**: *Subject: Stress levels at DEFCON 1*

- **Can't stop, won't stop sweating**: *Subject: Time to cool down, hotshot*

You get the drift. Symptoms are your body's way of saying, "Yo, brain! Pay attention! Something's going on down here!"

The Body... I Mean, the Email

Now, if symptoms are the subject lines, the actual messages are the, well, *messages*. The details. The nitty-gritty. And just like emails, these messages can range from super important ("Hey, your appendix is about to burst, FYI") to totally trivial ("You've got an itch. Yeah, just a regular itch. Nothing to see here.").

But here's where it gets tricky. Unlike emails, your body's messages aren't always crystal clear. Sometimes, they're downright cryptic. They're like those annoying emails from your boss that say stuff like, "We need to talk about your performance," and leave you wondering, "Am I getting a promotion or getting fired?!"

Spam Alert: When Noise Becomes Nonsense

Just like your inbox, your body can get flooded with spam. **False alarms, hypochondria, and straight-up weird stuff** that makes you go, "WTF, body?!"

The Boy Who Cried Wolf: False Alarms

Ever had a sudden, sharp pain that made you think, "This is it. I'm dying"? Only to have it disappear a minute later, leaving you feeling like a drama queen? Congrats, you've experienced a false alarm.

False alarms are like those emails that scream, "URGENT!!!!!", only for you to open them and find out they're just trying to sell you discount Viagra. * facepalm *

Dr. Google's Evil Twin: Hypochondria

Then there's hypochondria—the ultimate spammer. It's like that annoying friend who's always blowing up your inbox with chain emails and conspiracy theories. "Dude, I'm pretty sure this mole is cancer. I read about it on this sketchy website..."

Newsflash: Not every headache is a brain tumor, and not every stomach ache is appendicitis. Chill out, WebMD warriors.

WTF, Body?!: Weird Stuff

And finally, there's the just plain weird stuff. Like when you sneeze so hard you fart a little (it's called "snarting," look it up), or when you get a random, inexplicable craving for pickles and ice cream. Bodies are weird, man. Don't try to understand them.

Forward to Failure: Ignoring Symptoms

Alright, so we've established that your body is like an inbox, full of important messages, spam, and WTF moments. But what happens when you ignore those messages? **Spoiler alert**: Nothing good.

The Ostrich Approach: Sticking Your Head in the Sand

Ignoring symptoms is like ignoring emails from your bank. Sure, you might avoid some bad news for a while, but sooner or later, your account's gonna get frozen, and you're gonna be up shit creek without a paddle.

Same goes for your body. Ignore those "low battery" warnings long enough, and eventually, you'll crash. Hard.

The Domino Effect: How Little Problems Become Big Ones

Here's the thing about ignoring symptoms: **little problems don't stay little**. They grow. They fester. They turn into big, nasty, impossible-to-ignore problems.

It's like when you ignore a tiny crack in your windshield, and suddenly, you're driving through a hailstorm, and BAM! Your windshield shatters, and you're sitting there going, "Well, shit. I should've fixed that when it was just a tiny crack."

The Wake-Up Call: When Your Body Says "Enough!"

Eventually, if you ignore your body's messages long enough, it'll send you a wake-up call. A big, loud, smack-you-upside-the-head wake-up call. Think heart attack, stroke, or some other equally terrifying health crisis.

Moral of the story: Don't ignore your body's messages. Unless you want to end up in the ER, explaining to the doctor that you "just thought the chest pain would go away on its own."

The Motherboard: Your Cellular Software

Alright, tech-savvy troops, buckle up! We're about to dive deep into the inner workings of your biological hardware. Think of your body as the ultimate supercomputer—only instead of silicon chips and circuit boards, you're rocking cells and DNA. Welcome to **The Motherboard: Your Cellular Software**.

Hardwired for Success: Cellular Basics

Before we start debugging, let's get acquainted with the basics. Your body is made up of trillions of cells—tiny, living machines that keep you ticking. Think of them as the **pixels on your screen**, the **bits and bytes** of your biological code.

The Cellular Blueprint: DNA

At the heart of every cell is the **DNA**, your genetic blueprint. It's like the **source code** of your body, dictating everything from your eye color to your propensity for dad jokes. DNA is packed into **chromosomes**, which are like the **folders** on your hard drive, organizing all that genetic info.

The Control Center: The Nucleus

The **nucleus** is the **control center** of the cell—the **CPU**, if you will. It houses your DNA and directs all the cell's activities. Think of it as the **mission control** where all the big decisions are made.

The Power Plant: Mitochondria

Meet the **mitochondria**, the **power plants** of your cells. These little guys convert food into energy, keeping your cellular machinery humming along. They're like the **battery packs** that keep your body powered up and ready to go.

The Assembly Line: Ribosomes

Ribosomes are the **assembly lines** where proteins are made. They read the instructions from your DNA and churn out the proteins your body needs to function. Think of them as the **3D printers** of your cells, building essential components from scratch.

Updating Your OS: Epigenetics for Dummies

Alright, so we've got the basics down. Now let's talk about **epigenetics**—the **software updates** of your biological OS. Epigenetics is all about how your genes are **expressed**, not just what they are. It's like the **settings** on your computer that determine how your programs run.

The On/Off Switch: Gene Expression

Imagine your genes as **apps** on your phone. Some are always running in the background, while others only activate when you need them. **Epigenetics** is the **on/off switch** that controls which genes are active and which are dormant.

The Environmental Factor: Lifestyle Choices

Here's where it gets interesting: **your lifestyle choices** can influence your epigenetics. What you eat, how much you exercise, even your stress levels—all these factors can **toggle** your genetic switches. It's like **customizing** your OS settings to optimize performance.

The Good, the Bad, and the Ugly: Epigenetic Changes

Not all epigenetic changes are created equal. Some are **good**, like the ones that help you adapt to a healthier lifestyle. Others are **bad**, like the ones that increase your risk of disease. And then there are the **ugly** ones—the glitches that can lead to all sorts of health issues.

Debugging 101: Fixing Cellular Glitches

Now that we understand the basics of our cellular software, let's talk about **debugging**. Just like any complex system, your body is prone to **glitches**—little hiccups that can throw everything out of whack. But don't worry, we've got some **troubleshooting tips** to get you back on track.

The Error Message: Cellular Damage

Cellular damage is like the **error message** that pops up when something's gone wrong. It can be caused by all sorts of things—**free radicals**, **toxins**, even **wear and tear** from everyday living. Think of it as the **blue screen of death** for your cells.

The Patch: Antioxidants

Enter **antioxidants**—the **patches** that fix cellular damage. These little heroes neutralize free radicals and repair damaged cells, keeping your biological OS running smoothly. Think of them as the **system updates** that keep your body bug-free.

The Reboot: Cellular Regeneration

Sometimes, the best way to fix a glitch is to **reboot** the system. In your body, that means **cellular regeneration**—the process of replacing old, damaged cells with new ones. It's like hitting the **reset button** to give your body a fresh start.

The Backup Plan: Stem Cells

And then there are **stem cells**—the **backup files** of your biological OS. These versatile cells can transform into any type of cell your body needs, providing a **safety net** in case of major glitches. Think of them as the **cloud storage** that keeps your data safe and sound.

The Cellular Network: Communication and Coordination

Your cells don't operate in isolation—they're part of a vast **network**, communicating and coordinating to keep your body running like a well-oiled machine. Think of it as the **internet of things**, but for your biological systems.

The Messengers: Hormones

Hormones are the **messengers** that carry signals between cells. They're like the **emails** and **texts** that keep you connected, relaying important info and coordinating actions. Whether it's regulating your metabolism or controlling your mood, hormones are the **communication backbone** of your body.

The Signal Boosters: Neurotransmitters

Neurotransmitters are the **signal boosters** that amplify messages in your nervous system. They're like the **Wi-Fi extenders** that keep your connection strong, ensuring that signals get where they need to go. From controlling your movements to regulating your emotions, neurotransmitters play a crucial role in keeping your body in sync.

The Network Administrators: The Immune System

And finally, there's the **immune system**—the **network administrators** that keep your cellular network safe and secure. They're like the **IT department** that monitors for threats, fights off infections, and keeps your body's defenses strong. Think of them as the **firewall** that protects your biological OS from harm.

Metabolic Cache: Clearing Out the Junk

Alright, fellow techies, it's time to talk about the **metabolic cache**—the junk that clogs up your system and slows you down. Think of it as the **temp files** and **browser history** that bog down your computer. Just like clearing out those digital cobwebs can speed up your machine, clearing out your metabolic cache can boost your health and energy levels. So, let's dive in and start **spring cleaning** your biological hard drive.

Cache Full: When Metabolism Goes Rogue

Your metabolism is like the **operating system** of your body—it controls how you convert food into energy and how you store or burn fat. But sometimes, things go awry. Your metabolism gets **glitchy**, and suddenly, you're feeling sluggish, gaining weight, and wondering what the heck happened to your get-up-and-go.

The Slowdown: Metabolic Syndrome

Meet **metabolic syndrome**—the **system error** that wreaks havoc on your health. It's a cluster of conditions that include high blood pressure, high blood sugar, excess body fat around the waist, and abnormal cholesterol or triglyceride levels. Think of it as the **blue screen of death** for your metabolism.

The Sugar Rush: Insulin Resistance

One of the key players in metabolic syndrome is **insulin resistance**. This is when your cells stop responding properly to insulin, the hormone that helps regulate your blood sugar. It's like your cells are **ignoring your emails**, leaving you with a **backlog** of unread messages (aka sugar) in your bloodstream.

The Fat Trap: Obesity

And then there's **obesity**—the **storage overload** that happens when your body holds onto too much fat. It's like your hard drive is **maxed out**, leaving no room for new data and slowing down your entire system. Obesity is a major risk factor for all sorts of health issues, from heart disease to diabetes.

Delete Temp Files: Detoxing for Nerds

So, how do you clear out your metabolic cache and get your system running smoothly again? It's all about **detoxing**—giving your body a chance to **reset** and **reboot**. But forget the fancy juice cleanses and colonics. We're talking about **real, science-backed strategies** that actually work.

The Reboot: Fasting

Fasting is like hitting the **reset button** on your metabolism. By giving your body a break from digesting food, you allow it to focus on **cleaning house**—repairing cells, reducing inflammation, and burning stored fat. Think of it as the **system reboot** that clears out the cobwebs and gets you back to peak performance.

Intermittent Fasting: The Quick Fix

Intermittent fasting is a popular approach that involves cycling between periods of eating and fasting. It's like the **quick reboot** that doesn't require a full system shutdown. Whether you're doing the **16/8 method** (fasting for 16 hours, eating for 8) or the **5:2 diet** (eating normally for 5 days, fasting for 2), intermittent fasting can help **jumpstart** your metabolism and **clear out the junk**.

Extended Fasting: The Deep Clean

For a more **thorough cleanse**, consider **extended fasting**—going without food for several days or even weeks. This is like the **deep clean** that gets into every nook and cranny of your system. But be warned: extended fasting is **not for the faint of heart**. It requires careful planning and medical supervision to ensure you're doing it safely.

The Cleanse: Whole Foods Diet

Another way to detox your metabolism is by **cleaning up your diet**. Swap out the **processed junk** for **whole, nutrient-dense foods**. Think of it as **upgrading your software**—replacing the **buggy, outdated programs** with **streamlined, efficient apps**.

The Upgrade: Nutrient-Dense Foods

Nutrient-dense foods are like the **premium apps** that optimize your system. They're packed with vitamins, minerals, and antioxidants that **support your metabolism** and **clear out the junk**. We're talking fruits, veggies, lean proteins, and healthy fats—the **good stuff** that fuels your body and keeps it running smoothly.

The Downgrade: Processed Foods

On the other hand, **processed foods** are like the **shady apps** that slow down your system and clog it up with **malware**. They're loaded with sugar, unhealthy fats, and artificial ingredients that **mess with your metabolism** and **leave you feeling sluggish**. Ditch the **junk food** and give your body the **high-quality fuel** it deserves.

The Flush: Hydration

And let's not forget about **hydration**. Water is like the **system flush** that **clears out the pipes** and **keeps everything flowing smoothly**. It helps your body **eliminate toxins, regulate temperature**, and **transport nutrients** where they're needed.

The Gold Standard: Water

Water is the **gold standard** when it comes to hydration. It's **pure, simple, and effective**, with **no added sugars or artificial ingredients**. Aim for **8 glasses a day** to keep your system **running smoothly** and **clear out the metabolic cache**.

The Upgrade: Infused Water

For a **tasty twist**, try **infused water**. Add slices of fruit, veggies, or herbs to your H2O for a **flavor boost** that's **low in calories** and **high in nutrients**. It's like the **custom theme** that makes your **operating system** look and feel **even better**.

Defragging Your Diet: Food Hacks for Longevity

Alright, so we've talked about **clearing out the junk** and **upgrading your software**. Now let's dive into some **specific food hacks** that can **optimize your metabolism** and **boost your longevity**. Think of these as the **shortcuts** and **tricks** that **streamline your system** and **make your life easier**.

The Power-Up: Superfoods

Superfoods are like the **power-ups** in your favorite video game—they **boost your stats** and **give you an edge**. These **nutrient-packed** foods are **loaded with antioxidants, vitamins**, and **minerals** that **support your metabolism** and **keep your body running smoothly**.

The Green Machine: Leafy Greens

Leafy greens are the **ultimate power-up** for your metabolism. They're **packed with nutrients** like **vitamin K, vitamin C**, and **folate**, which **support your immune system, boost your energy levels**, and **keep your body in tip-top shape**. Load up on **spinach, kale**, and **collard greens** to **supercharge your system**.

The Berry Blast: Berries

Berries are like the **sweet treat** that's **actually good for you**. They're **loaded with antioxidants** that **fight inflammation**, **boost your immune system**, and **support your metabolism**. Whether you're snacking on **blueberries, strawberries**, or **raspberries**, you're giving your body a **delicious dose** of **health-boosting nutrients**.

The Fat Burner: Healthy Fats

Healthy fats are like the **high-octane fuel** that **keeps your engine running smoothly**. They **support your metabolism, boost your energy levels**, and **help you burn fat**. But not all fats are created equal—**steer clear** of the **trans fats** and **hydrogenated oils** that **clog up your system** and **slow you down**.

The Omega Boost: Omega-3s

Omega-3 fatty acids are the **ultimate fat burner**. They **reduce inflammation, support heart health**, and **boost your metabolism**. Load up on **fatty fish** like **salmon, mackerel**, and **sardines**, or **plant-based sources** like **chia seeds, flaxseeds**, and **walnuts** to **give your body** the **healthy fats** it needs.

The Avocado Advantage: Monounsaturated Fats

Monounsaturated fats are another **key player** in the **fat-burning game**. They **support heart health, boost your metabolism**, and **keep you feeling full** and **satisfied**. **Avocados** are a **top source** of these **healthy fats**, along with **olive oil, nuts**, and **seeds**.

The Protein Punch: Lean Proteins

Lean proteins are like the **building blocks** of your metabolism. They **support muscle growth, boost your energy**

levels, and **help you burn fat**. But **skip the red meat** and **processed junk—opt for** the **lean, clean proteins** that **fuel your body** without **weighing you down**.

The Plant Power: Plant-Based Proteins

Plant-based proteins are the **ultimate power punch** for your metabolism. They're **low in calories, high in nutrients**, and **packed with fiber** that **keeps you feeling full** and **satisfied**. Load up on **beans, lentils, tofu**, and **tempeh** to **give your body** the **plant-powered protein** it needs.

The Seafood Solution: Fish and Shellfish

Fish and **shellfish** are another **great source** of **lean protein**. They're **packed with nutrients** like **omega-3s, vitamin D**, and **selenium**, which **support your metabolism** and **keep your body running smoothly**. Opt for **sustainable seafood** options to **protect the planet** while **boosting your health**.

The Cloud: Your Brain on Tech

Alright, listen up, brainiacs! It's time to dive into the **ultimate control center** of your biological supercomputer—your brain. Think of it as the **cloud storage** where all your thoughts, memories, and emotions are stored. Just like any tech system, your brain needs some TLC to keep it running smoothly. So, let's **hack into** the mysteries of your noggin and **optimize** that gray matter.

Bandwidth Boost: Enhancing Brain Power

Your brain is like the **internet connection** of your body—it processes information, sends signals, and keeps everything running smoothly. But just like a slow internet connection, a sluggish brain can leave you feeling **frustrated** and **unproductive**. So, let's talk about **boosting your bandwidth** and **enhancing your brain power**.

The Brain Boosters: Nootropics

Nootropics are like the **turbo boost** for your brain—they **enhance cognitive function**, **improve memory**, and **increase focus**. Think of them as the **high-speed internet** that **keeps your connection strong** and **your brain running smoothly.**

The Caffeine Kick: Coffee and Tea

Caffeine is the **OG nootropic**—it's been **boosting brains** for centuries. Whether you're sipping on a **steaming cup of joe** or **enjoying a soothing cup of tea**, caffeine **increases alertness, improves focus**, and **keeps you on your toes**. Just **don't overdo it**—too much caffeine can leave you **jittery** and **anxious.**

The Herbal Helpers: Ginkgo Biloba and Bacopa Monnieri

Ginkgo biloba and **bacopa monnieri** are **herbal nootropics** that have been **used for centuries** to **boost brain power.** Ginkgo **improves blood flow** to the brain, **enhancing cognitive function**, while bacopa **supports memory** and **reduces anxiety.** Think of them as the **natural upgrades** that **keep your brain running smoothly.**

The Brain Food: Nutrients for Neurons

Your brain **runs on fuel**, just like any other part of your body. But not all fuel is created equal—some **nutrients** are **better for your brain** than others. So, let's talk about the **best brain food** to **keep your neurons firing** on all cylinders.

The Omega-3 Advantage: Fatty Fish

Omega-3 fatty acids are the **ultimate brain food**—they **support brain health, improve cognitive function**, and **reduce inflammation.** Load up on **fatty fish** like **salmon, mackerel**, and **sardines**, or **plant-based sources** like **chia seeds, flaxseeds**, and **walnuts** to **give your brain** the **healthy fats** it needs.

The Antioxidant Army: Berries and Leafy Greens

Antioxidants are like the **bodyguards** of your brain—they **protect your neurons** from **damage, reduce inflammation,** and **support cognitive function. Berries** and **leafy greens** are **packed with antioxidants**, so **load up** on these **brain-boosting foods** to **keep your mind sharp.**

Firewall Fundamentals: Protecting Mental Health

Just like your computer needs a **firewall** to **protect it from threats,** your brain needs **defenses** to **keep it safe** and **healthy.** Mental health is **crucial** for **optimal brain function,** so let's talk about **building a strong firewall** to **protect your mind.**

The Stress Busters: Mindfulness and Meditation

Stress is like the **malware** that **slows down your system** and **messes with your brain.** But **mindfulness** and **meditation** are the **antivirus software** that **keeps your mind clear** and **your brain running smoothly.** These **ancient practices reduce stress, improve focus,** and **boost mental health.**

The Mindful Moment: Living in the Now

Mindfulness is all about **living in the present moment**—it's the **art of paying attention** to what's happening **right now,** without **judgment** or **distraction.** By **practicing mindfulness,** you can **reduce stress, improve focus,** and **boost your mental health.** Think of it as the **system update** that **keeps your brain running smoothly.**

The Meditation Magic: Quieting the Mind

Meditation is like the **deep clean** for your mind—it **clears out the clutter, reduces stress,** and **boosts mental clarity.** Whether you're **sitting in silence** or **following a guided meditation,** this **ancient practice** can **transform your mental health** and **keep your brain running smoothly.**

The Social Network: Connections IRL

Social connections are like the **Wi-Fi signal** that **keeps your brain connected** and **running smoothly.** But in today's **digital age,** it's easy to **lose sight** of the **importance of IRL connections.** So, let's talk about **building a strong social network** to **support your mental health.**

The Friendship Factor: Quality over Quantity

Friendships are the **backbone** of your **social network**—they **provide support, reduce stress,** and **boost mental health.** But **quality** is more important than **quantity**—a **few close friends** can **make a bigger impact** on your **mental health** than a hundred acquaintances. So, **invest in your friendships** and **build a strong support system.**

The Community Connection: Finding Your Tribe

Community is like the **extended family** that **supports you, inspires you**, and **keeps you connected.** Whether it's a **local club**, a **volunteer group**, or an **online community, finding your tribe** can **boost your mental health** and **keep your brain running smoothly.**

Upgrading Your Hardware: Neuroplasticity and You

Your brain is like the **ultimate tech gadget**—it's **adaptable, upgradable**, and **always evolving.** This is thanks to **neuroplasticity**—the **ability of your brain** to **change, grow,** and **adapt** over time. So, let's talk about **upgrading your hardware** and **harnessing the power** of neuroplasticity.

The Learning Curve: Lifelong Education

Lifelong learning is like the **continuous upgrade** for your brain—it **keeps your mind sharp, boosts cognitive function,** and **supports neuroplasticity.** Whether you're **taking a class, reading a book**, or **learning a new skill, lifelong education** is the **key to a healthy brain.**

The Skill Set: Mastering New Abilities

Learning new skills is like the **software update** that **keeps your brain running smoothly.** Whether it's a **new language**, a **musical instrument**, or a **coding language, mastering new abilities** can **boost your brain power** and **support neuroplasticity.**

The Knowledge Quest: Exploring New Ideas

Exploring new ideas is like the **adventure** that **keeps your brain engaged** and **excited.** Whether you're **reading a book, watching a documentary**, or **attending a lecture,**

seeking out new knowledge can **expand your mind** and **support neuroplasticity.**

The Brain Gym: Exercise for Neurogenesis

Exercise is like the **workout** for your brain—it **boosts neurogenesis** (the **creation of new neurons**), **improves cognitive function**, and **supports mental health.** So, let's talk about **getting physical** and **giving your brain** the **workout** it needs.

The Cardio Kick: Aerobic Exercise

Aerobic exercise is like the **cardio session** that **gets your heart pumping** and your **brain firing** on all cylinders. Whether you're **running, cycling,** or **dancing, cardio** can **boost your brain power** and **support neurogenesis.**

The Strength Training: Resistance Exercise

Resistance exercise is like the **weightlifting session** that **builds your muscles** and **boosts your brain.** Whether you're **lifting weights, doing yoga,** or **practicing tai chi, strength training** can **improve cognitive function** and **support neuroplasticity.**

The Server Room: Heart Health Hacks

Alright, folks, it's time to talk about the **heart** of the matter—literally. Think of your heart as the **server room** of your body. It's the **central hub** that **keeps everything running smoothly**, pumping blood and oxygen to every corner of your biological supercomputer. But just like any server room, your heart needs some **serious TLC** to keep it in tip-top shape. So, let's dive in and **hack into** the secrets of heart health.

Optimizing Uptime: Keeping Your Heart Ticking

Your heart is like the **24/7 server** that **never takes a break**. It's **always on**, **always working**, and **always essential** to your survival. But just like any piece of tech, your heart can **wear out**, **glitch**, or even **crash** if you don't take care of it. So, let's talk about **optimizing uptime** and **keeping your heart ticking** strong.

The Heart-Healthy Diet: Fueling Your Engine

Just like a **server room** needs **clean, efficient fuel** to run smoothly, your heart needs a **healthy diet** to keep it **strong** and **resilient**. So, let's talk about the **best foods** to **fuel your heart** and **keep it running smoothly**.

The Mediterranean Magic: Olive Oil and Fish

The **Mediterranean diet** is like the **gold standard** for heart health. It's **packed with healthy fats, fresh produce**, and **lean proteins** that **support your heart** and **keep it running smoothly**. Load up on **olive oil, fatty fish** like **salmon** and **mackerel**, and **plenty of fruits and veggies** to **give your heart** the **fuel** it needs.

The Fiber Fix: Whole Grains and Legumes

Fiber is like the **system cleaner** that **keeps your heart** running smoothly. It **lowers cholesterol, improves digestion,**

and **supports heart health.** Load up on **whole grains** like **oats, brown rice,** and **quinoa,** and **legumes** like **beans, lentils,** and **chickpeas** to **give your heart** the **fiber boost** it needs.

The Heart-Healthy Lifestyle: Habits for a Strong Ticker

A **healthy lifestyle** is like the **preventive maintenance** that **keeps your server room** running smoothly. It's all about the **habits** and **routines** that **support your heart** and **keep it in tip-top shape.** So, let's talk about the **best habits** for a **strong, healthy heart.**

The Exercise Equation: Getting Your Heart Pumping

Exercise is like the **regular reboot** that **keeps your heart** running smoothly. It **strengthens your heart muscle, improves circulation,** and **boosts your overall health.** Whether you're **running, cycling, swimming,** or **dancing, getting your heart pumping** is **essential** for **optimal heart health.**

The Sleep Solution: Rest and Recovery

Sleep is like the **nightly backup** that **keeps your heart** running smoothly. It **reduces stress, supports heart health,** and **keeps your body** in **tip-top shape.** Aim for **7-9 hours** of **quality sleep** each night to **give your heart** the **rest** it needs.

Load Balancing: Stress Management

Stress is like the **system overload** that **slows down your server** and **messes with your heart.** It **increases blood pressure, strains your heart,** and **leads to all sorts of health issues.** But with the **right strategies,** you can **manage stress** and **keep your heart** running smoothly. So, let's talk about **load balancing** and **stress management.**

The Mind-Body Connection: Holistic Health

Your **mind** and **body** are like the **interconnected systems** that **work together** to **keep you healthy**. When one is **stressed**, the other **feels the strain**. So, let's talk about the **holistic approaches** that **support your heart** and **keep your mind and body** in **sync**.

The Yoga Yin: Flexibility and Flow

Yoga is like the **flexibility training** that **keeps your mind and body** in **sync**. It **reduces stress, improves flexibility,** and **supports heart health.** Whether you're a **beginner** or a **seasoned yogi, incorporating yoga** into your **routine** can **boost your heart health** and **keep you feeling** your **best**.

The Tai Chi Tango: Balance and Harmony

Tai chi is like the **dance of balance** that **keeps your mind and body** in **harmony**. It **reduces stress, improves balance,** and **supports heart health.** This **ancient practice** is a **gentle, low-impact way** to **boost your heart health** and **keep you feeling** your **best**.

The Breathing Break: Mindful Moments

Breathing exercises are like the **quick reboot** that **clears your mind** and **reduces stress**. They **calm your nervous system, lower your blood pressure,** and **support heart health.** So, let's talk about the **best breathing techniques** to **keep your heart** running smoothly.

The 4-7-8 Technique: Calm and Collected

The **4-7-8 breathing technique** is like the **instant calm** that **reduces stress** and **supports heart health.** Here's how it works: **inhale** for **4 seconds, hold your breath** for **7 seconds,** and **exhale** for **8 seconds.** Repeat this **cycle** for a **few minutes** to **feel the calming effects** and **boost your heart health.**

The Box Breathing: Balance and Focus

Box breathing is like the **balancing act** that **keeps your mind** and **body** in **sync**. Here's how it works: **inhale** for **4 seconds**, **hold your breath** for **4 seconds**, **exhale** for **4 seconds**, and **hold your breath** again for **4 seconds**. Repeat this **cycle** for a **few minutes** to **feel the balancing effects** and **boost your heart health**.

Avoiding Downtime: Preventing Heart Disease

Heart disease is like the **system crash** that **shuts down your server** and **leaves you scrambling**. It's a **serious issue** that **affects millions** of Americans each year. But with the **right strategies**, you can **prevent heart disease** and **keep your heart** running smoothly. So, let's talk about **avoiding downtime** and **preventing heart disease**.

The Risk Factors: Know Your Enemy

To **prevent heart disease**, you need to **know your enemy**. Understanding the **risk factors** can **help you make informed decisions** and **keep your heart** in **tip-top shape**. So, let's talk about the **most common risk factors** for heart disease.

The High Blood Pressure: The Silent Killer

High blood pressure is like the **silent killer** that **strains your heart** and **leads to heart disease**. It's often **symptomless**, making it **difficult to detect**. But with **regular check-ups** and **lifestyle changes**, you can **manage your blood pressure** and **keep your heart** running smoothly.

The High Cholesterol: The Clogged Pipes

High cholesterol is like the **clogged pipes** that **slow down your system** and **lead to heart disease**. It **builds up in your arteries, restricting blood flow** and **straining your heart**. But with a **healthy diet** and **regular exercise**, you can **manage your cholesterol** and **keep your heart** running smoothly.

The Preventive Measures: Keeping Your Heart Healthy

Preventing heart disease is all about the **proactive measures** that **keep your heart** in **tip-top shape**. It's about **making smart choices**, **staying informed**, and **taking control** of your health. So, let's talk about the **best preventive measures** to **keep your heart** running smoothly.

The Regular Check-Ups: Staying Informed

Regular check-ups are like the **system updates** that **keep your heart** running smoothly. They **help you stay informed** about your **health status** and **catch any issues** early. Schedule **regular appointments** with your **doctor** to **monitor your heart health** and **make any necessary adjustments**.

The Lifestyle Changes: Making Smart Choices

Lifestyle changes are like the **software upgrades** that **keep your heart** running smoothly. They **improve your overall health** and **reduce your risk** of heart disease. Whether it's **quitting smoking**, **eating healthier**, or **exercising more**, **making smart choices** can **boost your heart health** and **keep you feeling** your **best**.

The Network: Social Connections IRL

Alright, folks, it's time to talk about the **ultimate social network**—the one that exists **IRL** (in real life), not just on your screen. Think of your social connections as the **Wi-Fi** that **keeps you connected**, **supported**, and **thriving**. Just like a strong internet connection, a strong social network can **boost your health**, **improve your well-being**, and **make life a whole lot more enjoyable**. So, let's dive in and **hack into** the secrets of building and maintaining **meaningful social connections**.

Router Reset: Revitalizing Relationships

Just like your Wi-Fi router sometimes needs a **reset** to **clear out the cobwebs** and **get back to peak performance**, your relationships can benefit from a **refresh** every now and then. So, let's talk about **revitalizing your relationships** and **keeping your social network** strong and vibrant.

The Friendship Factor: Quality over Quantity

When it comes to friendships, **quality** is way more important than **quantity**. Having a **few close friends** who **get you**, **support you**, and **make you laugh** is **worth more** than a **hundred acquaintances** who **barely know your name**. So, let's talk about **building strong, meaningful friendships** that **stand the test of time**.

The BFF Blueprint: Building Strong Bonds

Building strong friendships is like **constructing a sturdy house**—it takes **time**, **effort**, and **the right materials**. Here are some **tips** for **building strong bonds** that **last**:

- **Be Present:** Show up for your friends, both **physically** and **emotionally. Listen** to them, **support** them, and **be there** when they need you.

- **Communicate**: Open, honest communication is the **key** to any strong relationship. **Share** your thoughts, **feelings**, and **experiences** with your friends, and **encourage them** to do the same.

- **Have Fun**: Don't forget to **laugh, play,** and **have fun** together. **Shared experiences** and **memories** are the **glue** that **holds friendships together.**

The Friendship Maintenance: Keeping Bonds Strong

Maintaining strong friendships is like **regularly updating your software**—it keeps things **running smoothly** and **prevents glitches**. Here are some **tips** for **keeping your bonds strong**:

- **Stay in Touch**: Regular communication is **key** to keeping friendships alive. **Text, call,** or **meet up** with your friends **regularly** to **stay connected**.

- **Be There**: Show up for your friends in **times of need**. Whether it's a **shoulder to cry on** or a **helping hand, being there** for your friends **strengthens your bond**.

- **Celebrate**: Celebrate your friends' **achievements, milestones**, and **just because. Sharing joy** and **happiness** is a **great way** to **keep your friendship strong**.

The Family Factor: Strengthening Ties

Family relationships can be **complicated, challenging,** and **downright messy** at times. But they're also some of the **most important connections** in our lives. So, let's talk about **strengthening family ties** and **keeping those bonds strong**.

The Family Blueprint: Building Strong Relationships

Building strong family relationships is like **planting a garden**—it takes **time**, **care**, and **patience**. Here are some **tips** for **strengthening family ties**:

- **Communicate**: Open, honest communication is **key** to strong family relationships. **Share** your thoughts, **feelings**, and **experiences** with your family, and **encourage them** to do the same.

- **Spend Time Together**: Quality time is **essential** for building strong family bonds. **Plan activities, outings**, or just **hang out** together to **strengthen your connections**.

- **Support Each Other**: Be there for your family in **times of need**. Whether it's a **shoulder to cry on** or a **helping hand, supporting each other** strengthens your **family bonds**.

The Family Maintenance: Keeping Relationships Strong

Maintaining strong family relationships is like **regularly tending to your garden**—it keeps things **growing** and **thriving**. Here are some **tips** for **keeping your family bonds strong**:

- **Stay Connected**: Regular communication is **key** to keeping family relationships alive. **Text, call,** or **visit** your family **regularly** to **stay connected**.

- **Resolve Conflicts**: Conflicts are **inevitable** in any relationship, but **resolving them** in a **healthy, constructive way** can **strengthen your bonds. Listen, communicate**, and **work together** to find **solutions**.

- **Celebrate**: Celebrate your family's **achievements, milestones**, and **just**

because. Sharing joy and **happiness** is a **great way** to **keep your family bonds strong.**

Ping of Loneliness: The Impact of Isolation

Loneliness is like the **ping** that **keeps coming back, reminding you** that something's **missing**. It's the **feeling of disconnection, isolation,** and **longing** for **meaningful social interactions.** And it's a **serious issue** that **affects millions** of Americans. So, let's talk about the **impact of loneliness** and **what you can do** to **combat it.**

The Loneliness Epidemic: A Growing Problem

Loneliness is a **growing epidemic** in our **fast-paced, digitally-connected** world. Despite being **more connected than ever,** many of us **feel more isolated** than ever. So, let's talk about the **causes** and **consequences** of loneliness.

The Causes: Why We Feel Lonely

Loneliness can be **caused** by a **variety of factors,** including:

- **Lack of Social Connections**: Not having enough **meaningful social interactions** can lead to **feelings of loneliness** and **isolation.**

- **Life Transitions**: Major life changes, such as **moving, changing jobs,** or **losing a loved one,** can **trigger feelings of loneliness.**

- **Social Anxiety**: Fear of **social situations** or **judgment** can **prevent us** from **forming meaningful connections,** leading to **loneliness.**

The Consequences: The Impact of Loneliness

Loneliness can have **serious consequences** for our **physical** and **mental health,** including:

- **Depression and Anxiety**: Loneliness is **strongly linked** to **depression** and **anxiety**, as well as other **mental health issues**.

- **Physical Health Problems**: Chronic loneliness can **increase the risk** of **heart disease, high blood pressure**, and **weakened immune system**.

- **Reduced Lifespan**: Studies have shown that **chronic loneliness** can **shorten lifespan** as much as **smoking** or **obesity**.

The Loneliness Antidote: Combating Isolation

Combating loneliness is like **finding the antidote** to a **poison**—it **requires effort, determination**, and **the right strategies**. So, let's talk about **effective ways** to **combat loneliness** and **build meaningful social connections**.

The Social Prescription: Building Connections

Building social connections is like **filling a prescription**—it **requires the right ingredients** and **dosage** to be **effective**. Here are some **tips** for **building meaningful connections**:

- **Join a Club or Group**: Find a **club, group,** or **activity** that **aligns with your interests** and **join in**. This is a **great way** to **meet like-minded people** and **form connections**.

- **Volunteer**: Volunteering is a **great way** to **meet new people** and **form meaningful connections** while **giving back** to your **community**.

- **Reach Out**: Don't be **afraid** to **reach out** to **friends, family,** or **acquaintances. Initiating contact** can **lead to meaningful connections** and **combat loneliness**.

The Self-Care Solution: Taking Care of Yourself

Taking care of yourself is like **applying a bandage** to a wound—it **helps heal** and **protect** you from **further harm.** Here are some **self-care tips** to **combat loneliness**:

- **Practice Mindfulness**: Mindfulness practices like **meditation** and **yoga** can **help reduce feelings of loneliness** and **improve mental health.**

- **Exercise**: Regular exercise **boosts mood, reduces stress**, and **improves overall well-being, combating feelings of loneliness.**

- **Seek Professional Help**: If feelings of loneliness are **persistent** and **affecting your daily life, consider seeking help** from a **mental health professional.**

Social DDoS Attacks: Dealing with Toxic People

Just like your computer can be **targeted by malicious attacks**, your social network can be **infiltrated by toxic people.** These **negative influences** can **drain your energy, damage your self-esteem**, and **wreak havoc** on your **mental health.** So, let's talk about **dealing with toxic people** and **protecting your social network.**

The Toxic Types: Identifying Negative Influences

Toxic people come in **all shapes and sizes**, but they **share some common traits.** Here are some **types** of **toxic people** to **watch out for**:

- **The Critic**: Always **finding fault** and **putting you down,** the **critic** can **damage your self-esteem** and **leave you feeling inadequate.**

- **The Drama Queen/King**: Constantly **creating drama** and **stirring up trouble,** the **drama queen/king** can **exhaust you** and **leave you feeling stressed.**

- **The Manipulator**: Using **guilt**, **shame**, or **other tactics** to **control you**, the **manipulator** can **leave you feeling trapped** and **powerless**.

The Defense Mechanisms: Protecting Yourself

Dealing with toxic people is like **installing a firewall**—it **requires strategies** and **tactics** to **protect yourself** and **keep your social network safe**. Here are some **tips** for **dealing with toxic people**:

- **Set Boundaries**: Establish **clear boundaries** and **stick to them. Communicate** your **needs** and **limits** to **toxic people** and **don't be afraid** to **say no**.

- **Limit Contact**: Reduce your **interactions** with **toxic people** as much as **possible. Limit contact** to **protect your mental health** and **well-being**.

- **Seek Support**: Talk to **trusted friends, family**, or a **mental health professional** about your **experiences** with **toxic people. Seeking support** can **help you cope** and **find solutions**.

The Power Supply: Energy Management

Alright, folks, it's time to talk about the **power supply** of your biological supercomputer—your **energy levels**. Think of your energy as the **battery life** of your body. Just like your smartphone, you need a **steady supply of power** to keep you **running smoothly** and **performing at your best**. So, let's dive in and **hack into** the secrets of **energy management**.

Battery Saver Mode: Balancing Rest and Activity

Your body is like a **high-performance device** that **needs both rest** and **activity** to **function optimally**. Too much of one or the other can **drain your battery** and leave you **feeling sluggish**. So, let's talk about **balancing rest and activity** to **keep your energy levels** high and **your body** running smoothly.

The Recharge Cycle: The Importance of Sleep

Sleep is like the **nightly recharge** that **keeps your battery** full and **your body** running smoothly. It's the **time** when your body **repairs, rejuvenates**, and **prepares** for the next day. So, let's talk about the **importance of sleep** and **how to get the most** out of your **recharge cycle**.

The Sleep Stages: Understanding Your Recharge

Your sleep is divided into **stages**, each with its own **unique benefits**. Understanding these **stages** can help you **optimize your sleep** and **maximize your energy levels**.

- **Stage 1: Light Sleep**: This is the **transition** from **wakefulness** to **sleep**. It's a **brief stage** where your **body relaxes** and **prepares** for deeper sleep.

- **Stage 2: Deeper Sleep**: During this stage, your **heart rate slows, body temperature drops**, and your **body prepares** for **deep sleep**.

- **Stage 3: Deep Sleep**: This is the **most restorative stage** of sleep. Your **body repairs tissues, boosts your immune system**, and **rejuvenates** your **brain**.

- **REM Sleep: Dream Time**: During REM (Rapid Eye Movement) sleep, your **brain processes information, consolidates memories**, and **prepares you** for the day ahead.

The Sleep Hygiene: Tips for Better Sleep

Good sleep hygiene is like the **maintenance routine** that **keeps your battery** in **top shape**. Here are some **tips** for **improving your sleep** and **boosting your energy levels**:

- **Consistent Schedule**: Go to **bed** and **wake up** at the **same time** every day, even on **weekends**. This **consistency** helps **regulate your internal clock** and **improve sleep quality**.

- **Create a Routine**: Establish a **bedtime routine** that **signals** to your **body** it's time to **sleep**. This could include **reading, taking a warm bath,** or **listening to calming music**.

- **Optimize Your Environment**: Make your **sleep environment** as **comfortable** and **conducive to sleep** as possible. This includes a **cool temperature, dark room**, and **comfortable bed**.

The Activity Boost: The Importance of Exercise

Exercise is like the **power boost** that **keeps your battery** charged and **your body** running smoothly. It **increases energy levels, improves mood**, and **enhances overall**

health. So, let's talk about the **importance of exercise** and **how to get the most** out of your **activity boost.**

The Exercise Types: Finding Your Fit

There are **many types** of exercise, each with its own **unique benefits.** Finding the **right fit** for you can **help you stay motivated** and **maximize your energy levels.**

- **Aerobic Exercise**: Activities like **running, cycling,** and **swimming** get your **heart pumping** and **boost your cardiovascular health.** They also **release endorphins,** the **feel-good hormones** that **improve mood** and **reduce stress.**

- **Strength Training**: Lifting **weights,** doing **bodyweight exercises,** or practicing **yoga** builds **muscle** and **improves strength.** It also **boosts metabolism,** helping you **burn more calories** even when you're **not exercising.**

- **Flexibility and Balance**: Activities like **yoga, tai chi,** and **stretching** improve **flexibility** and **balance,** helping you **move more efficiently** and **reduce the risk of injury.**

The Exercise Hacks: Tips for Staying Active

Staying active is like the **regular maintenance** that **keeps your battery** charged and **your body** running smoothly. Here are some **tips** for **incorporating exercise** into your **daily routine** and **boosting your energy levels:**

- **Find What You Love**: Choose activities that you **enjoy** and **look forward to.** Whether it's **dancing, hiking,** or **playing a sport,** finding what you **love** makes it **easier to stay motivated.**

- **Mix It Up**: Variety is the **spice of life**, and it's also the **key to staying active**. Mix up your **exercise routine** to **keep things interesting** and **challenge your body** in new ways.

- **Make It a Habit**: Incorporate exercise into your **daily routine** so it becomes a **habit**. Whether it's a **morning walk**, a **lunchtime workout**, or an **evening yoga session**, making exercise a **habit** helps you **stay consistent**.

Overclocking: The Dangers of Burnout

Just like **overclocking** your computer can **push it beyond its limits** and **cause it to crash**, pushing your body **too hard** can lead to **burnout**. Burnout is like the **system overload** that **drains your battery, leaves you feeling exhausted**, and **can even lead to serious health issues**. So, let's talk about the **dangers of burnout** and **how to avoid it**.

The Burnout Symptoms: Recognizing the Signs

Recognizing the **signs of burnout** is like **spotting the warning signs** that your **system** is about to **crash**. Here are some **common symptoms** of burnout:

- **Chronic Fatigue**: Feeling **constantly tired**, even after **rest**. This is a **sign** that your **body** is **overworked** and **needs a break**.

- **Loss of Motivation**: Losing **interest** in things you **used to enjoy**. This can **indicate** that you're **overwhelmed** and **need to recharge**.

- **Increased Irritability**: Feeling **more irritable** or **short-tempered** than usual. This is a **sign** that your **body** is **under stress** and **needs a break**.

The Burnout Prevention: Strategies for Staying Balanced

Preventing burnout is like **installing a cooling system** to **keep your computer** running smoothly and **avoid overheating.** Here are some **strategies** for **staying balanced** and **avoiding burnout:**

- **Set Boundaries:** Establish **clear boundaries** between **work** and **personal time.** This **helps you avoid** feeling **overwhelmed** and **gives you time** to **recharge.**

- **Prioritize Self-Care:** Make **self-care** a **priority.** This includes **getting enough sleep, eating well,** and **taking time** for **relaxation** and **hobbies.**

- **Learn to Say No:** Don't be **afraid** to **say no** to **tasks** or **commitments** that **overwhelm you.** It's **okay** to **set limits** and **protect your energy.**

Energy Efficiency: Maximizing Your Output

Just like a **well-optimized computer** can **run more efficiently** and **get more done** with **less energy,** a **well-optimized body** can **maximize your output** and **help you achieve more** with **less effort.** So, let's talk about **energy efficiency** and **how to get the most** out of your **power supply.**

The Nutrition Factor: Fueling Your Body

Nutrition is like the **fuel** that **keeps your body** running smoothly. The **right foods** can **boost your energy levels, improve your mood,** and **help you perform** at your **best.** So, let's talk about the **best foods** for **maximizing your energy.**

The Energy Boosters: Foods for Fuel

Some foods are **better** than others when it comes to **boosting your energy levels.** Here are some **energy-boosting foods** to **incorporate** into your **diet:**

- **Complex Carbohydrates**: Foods like **whole grains, fruits**, and **vegetables** provide **sustained energy** and **keep you feeling full** and **satisfied**.

- **Lean Proteins**: Foods like **chicken, fish, beans,** and **nuts** provide the **building blocks** your **body needs** to **repair** and **rejuvenate**.

- **Healthy Fats**: Foods like **avocados, nuts,** and **seeds** provide **essential fats** that **support brain function** and **boost energy levels**.

The Hydration Hack: Staying Hydrated

Hydration is like the **oil** that **keeps your body** running smoothly. Staying **well-hydrated** can **boost your energy levels, improve your mood**, and **help you perform** at your **best**. Here are some **tips** for **staying hydrated**:

- **Drink Water Regularly**: Aim for **8 glasses** of **water** a day to **keep your body** well-hydrated.

- **Eat Hydrating Foods**: Foods like **fruits** and **vegetables** are **high in water content** and **can help keep you hydrated**.

- **Avoid Dehydrating Drinks**: Limit your **intake** of **caffeine** and **alcohol**, as they **can** dehydrate you.

The Mindset Shift: The Power of Positive Thinking

Your **mindset** is like the **software** that **controls your body**. A **positive mindset** can **boost your energy levels, improve your mood**, and **help you perform** at your **best**. So, let's talk about the **power of positive thinking** and **how to shift your mindset**.

The Gratitude Practice: Focusing on the Good

Gratitude is like the **antivirus software** that **protects your mind** from **negative thoughts** and **boosts your energy levels**. Here are some **tips** for **practicing gratitude**:

- **Keep a Gratitude Journal**: Write down **three things** you're **grateful for** each day. This **helps you focus** on the **positive aspects** of your life and **boosts your mood**.

- **Express Gratitude**: Tell the **people in your life** how **grateful** you are for them. This **strengthens your relationships** and **boosts your energy levels**.

- **Reframe Negative Thoughts**: When you **catch yourself** thinking **negatively**, try to **reframe** those thoughts in a **positive light**. This **helps you stay focused** on the **good** and **keeps your energy levels high**.

The Mindfulness Moment: Staying Present

Mindfulness is like the **system update** that **keeps your mind** running smoothly and **helps you stay present**. Here are some **tips** for **practicing mindfulness**:

- **Focus on the Present**: Pay **attention** to what's happening **right now**, without **judgment** or **distraction**. This **helps you stay grounded** and **reduces stress**.

- **Practice Meditation**: Meditation is a **great way** to **cultivate mindfulness** and **reduce stress**. Even a **few minutes** a day can **make a big difference**.

- **Engage Your Senses**: Use your **senses** to **stay present**. Notice the **sights, sounds, smells, tastes,** and **textures** around you. This **helps you stay connected** to the **present moment**.

The Upgrade Cycle: Habits for Longevity

Alright, folks, it's time to talk about the **upgrade cycle**—the **habits** and **routines** that **keep your body** running smoothly and **boost your longevity**. Think of your habits as the **software updates** that **optimize your system, fix bugs**, and **enhance performance**. So, let's dive in and **hack into** the secrets of **habits for longevity**.

Patch Notes: Tracking Your Progress

Just like a **software developer** keeps **detailed records** of **changes** and **improvements**, tracking your **progress** is **essential** for **optimizing your habits** and **boosting your longevity**. So, let's talk about the **importance of tracking** and **how to do it effectively**.

The Progress Tracker: Tools for Success

Tracking your **progress** is like **keeping a log** of your **updates** and **improvements**. It **helps you stay accountable, identify patterns**, and **make informed decisions**. Here are some **tools** for **tracking your progress**:

The Journal Method: Writing It Down

Journaling is like the **old-school** way of **tracking your progress**. It's **simple, effective**, and **allows you** to **reflect** on your **journey**. Here are some **tips** for **journaling**:

- **Daily Entries**: Write down your **thoughts, feelings**, and **experiences** each day. This **helps you stay connected** to your **goals** and **track your progress**.

- **Reflective Questions**: Ask yourself **reflective questions** like, "What did I learn today?" or "What can I do better tomorrow?" This **helps you stay focused** and **make improvements**.

- **Gratitude Practice**: Include a **gratitude section** in your journal to **focus on the positive** and **boost your mood**.

The App Approach: Digital Tracking

Apps are like the **modern** way of **tracking your progress**. They're **convenient, user-friendly**, and **packed with features** to **help you stay on track**. Here are some **tips** for **using apps**:

- **Choose the Right App**: Find an app that **meets your needs** and **supports your goals**. Whether it's a **fitness tracker**, a **food diary**, or a **habit tracker**, the **right app** can **make a big difference**.

- **Set Reminders**: Use the app's **reminder feature** to **keep you on track** and **ensure you don't miss** any **important tasks**.

- **Analyze Data**: Many apps **provide data analysis** to **help you identify patterns** and **make informed decisions**. Use this **information** to **optimize your habits** and **boost your longevity**.

The Goal Setting: Aiming for Success

Setting **goals** is like **defining the scope** of your **software update**. It **helps you stay focused, motivated**, and **on track** to **achieve your objectives**. So, let's talk about **effective goal setting** and **how to stay motivated**.

The SMART Goals: Specific, Measurable, Achievable, Relevant, Time-Bound

SMART goals are like the **blueprint** for your **success**. They **provide a clear roadmap** and **help you stay focused** on your **objectives**. Here's how to **set SMART goals**:

- **Specific**: Make your goals **clear** and **specific**. Instead of saying, "I want to exercise more," say, "I will exercise for 30 minutes, three times a week."

- **Measurable**: Ensure your goals are **measurable** so you can **track your progress**. For example, "I will lose 10 pounds in three months."

- **Achievable**: Set goals that are **realistic** and **achievable**. Don't set yourself up for **failure** by aiming too high.

- **Relevant**: Make sure your goals are **relevant** to your **overall objectives**. They should **align** with your **values** and **priorities**.

- **Time-Bound**: Give your goals a **deadline** to **keep you motivated** and **on track**. For example, "I will complete a 5k run by the end of the month."

The Motivation Boost: Staying on Track

Staying **motivated** is like the **fuel** that **keeps you going** on your **journey** to **longevity**. Here are some **tips** for **boosting your motivation**:

- **Visualize Success**: Imagine yourself **achieving your goals**. This **helps you stay focused** and **motivated**.

- **Celebrate Milestones**: Celebrate your **achievements**, no matter how small. This **keeps you motivated** and **on track**.

- **Find Support**: Surround yourself with **people who support** your **goals** and **encourage you** to **keep going**.

Beta Testing: Trying New Routines

Just like **beta testing** a **new software update**, trying **new routines** is **essential** for **optimizing your habits** and **boosting your longevity**. So, let's talk about the **importance of experimenting** and **how to do it effectively**.

The Experimentation Phase: Exploring New Habits

Experimenting with **new habits** is like **testing different features** in a **software update**. It **helps you find** what **works best** for you and **optimize your routines**. Here are some **tips** for **experimenting with new habits**:

- **Start Small**: Begin with **small changes** and **gradually build** on them. This **makes it easier** to **stick to new habits** and **see results**.

- **Track Results**: Keep a **record** of your **experiments** and **track the results**. This **helps you identify** what **works** and what **doesn't**.

- **Adjust as Needed**: Don't be **afraid** to **make adjustments** based on your **results. Tweaking your habits** can **help you find** the **perfect routine** for you.

The Feedback Loop: Learning from Experience

The **feedback loop** is like the **continuous improvement cycle** that **helps you refine** your **habits** and **optimize your routines**. It **involves observing, analyzing,** and **adjusting** based on your **experiences**. Here are some **tips** for **using the feedback loop**:

- **Observe**: Pay **attention** to how your **new habits** are **affecting you**. Notice any **changes** in your **energy levels, mood,** and **overall well-being**.

- **Analyze**: Reflect on your **observations** and **analyze** the **results**.

What **worked** well? What **didn't**? What **changes** do you **need to make**?

- **Adjust**: Based on your **analysis**, make **adjustments** to your **habits**. This **helps you** **refine** your **routines** and **optimize your results**.

Version Control: Maintaining Healthy Habits

Just like **version control** in **software development**, maintaining **healthy habits** is **essential** for **long-term success** and **longevity**. So, let's talk about the **importance of consistency** and **how to stay on track**.

The Consistency Key: Sticking to Your Habits

Consistency is like the **backbone** of your **habits**. It **keeps you on track, helps you achieve your goals**, and **ensures long-term success**. Here are some **tips** for **maintaining consistency**:

- **Create a Routine**: Establish a **daily routine** that **incorporates** your **healthy habits**. This **makes it easier** to **stick to them** and **stay consistent**.

- **Set Reminders**: Use **reminders** to **keep you on track**. Whether it's a **calendar alert**, a **phone notification**, or a **sticky note, reminders** can **help you stay consistent**.

- **Make It a Habit**: Turn your **healthy habits** into **automatic behaviors**. The **more you practice**, the **easier it becomes** to **stick to them**.

The Relapse Plan: Dealing with Setbacks

Setbacks are like the **bugs** in your **software update**—they **happen**, but they **don't have to derail** your **progress**. Having a **relapse plan** can **help you stay on track** and **bounce**

back from **setbacks**. Here are some **tips** for **dealing with setbacks**:

- **Identify Triggers**: Recognize the **triggers** that **lead to setbacks**. This **helps you avoid** them and **stay on track**.

- **Have a Plan**: Develop a **plan** for **dealing with setbacks**. This **could include seeking support, adjusting your habits**, or **taking a break** to **recharge**.

- **Learn from Mistakes**: Use **setbacks** as **learning opportunities**. Reflect on what **went wrong** and **how you can improve** in the **future**.

The Firewall: Immune System Boost

Alright, folks, it's time to talk about the **ultimate defense system** of your biological supercomputer—your **immune system**. Think of it as the **firewall** that **protects you** from **invasions**, **keeps you healthy**, and **ensures your body** runs smoothly. Just like any tech system, your immune system needs some **serious TLC** to keep it in tip-top shape. So, let's dive in and **hack into** the secrets of **boosting your immune system**.

Antivirus Software: Preventing Illness

Your immune system is like the **antivirus software** that **protects your body** from **harmful invaders**. It **identifies**, **neutralizes**, and **eliminates** threats, keeping you **healthy** and **strong**. So, let's talk about **preventing illness** and **keeping your immune system** in **top shape**.

The Germ Busters: Hygiene Habits

Good hygiene is like the **first line of defense** against **germs** and **viruses**. It **keeps you clean, healthy**, and **protected**. So, let's talk about the **best hygiene habits** to **boost your immune system**.

The Handwashing Ritual: Keeping Germs at Bay

Handwashing is like the **daily maintenance** that **keeps your system** running smoothly. It **removes germs, prevents illness**, and **keeps you healthy**. Here are some **tips** for **effective handwashing**:

- **Use Soap and Water**: Wash your hands with **soap** and **warm water** for at least **20 seconds**. This **helps remove germs** and **keeps your hands clean**.

- **Scrub Thoroughly**: Make sure to **scrub** all parts of your hands, including **between your fingers** and **under your nails**. This **ensures** you **remove all germs**.

- **Dry Completely**: Dry your hands **thoroughly** with a **clean towel**. This **helps prevent** the **spread of germs**.

The Cleanliness Crusade: Keeping Surfaces Germ-Free

Cleaning surfaces is like the **regular update** that **keeps your system** free of **bugs** and **viruses**. It **removes germs, prevents illness**, and **keeps your environment** healthy. Here are some **tips** for **keeping surfaces clean**:

- **Use Disinfectants**: Use **disinfectant wipes** or **sprays** to **clean surfaces** regularly. This **helps remove germs** and **keeps your environment clean**.

- **Focus on High-Touch Areas**: Pay **special attention** to **high-touch areas** like **doorknobs, light switches**, and **countertops**. These areas **harbor the most germs**.

- **Wash Cloths and Sponges**: Regularly **wash** your **cleaning cloths** and **sponges** to **prevent** the **spread of germs**.

The Nutrition Boost: Foods for Immunity

Nutrition is like the **fuel** that **keeps your immune system** running smoothly. The **right foods** can **boost your immunity, improve your health**, and **keep you protected** from **illness**. So, let's talk about the **best foods** for **boosting your immune system**.

The Vitamin C Squad: Citrus Fruits and More

Vitamin C is like the **superhero** of your **immune system**. It **boosts immunity, fights infections**, and **keeps you healthy**. Here are some **foods** that are **packed with vitamin C**:

- **Citrus Fruits**: Oranges, **lemons, limes,** and **grapefruits** are **loaded with vitamin C.** They **boost your immunity** and **keep you healthy**.

- **Berries**: Berries like **strawberries, blueberries,** and **raspberries** are **rich in vitamin C** and **antioxidants**. They **support your immune system** and **keep you strong**.

- **Bell Peppers**: Bell peppers are **packed with vitamin C** and **other nutrients** that **boost your immunity.**

The Antioxidant Army: Colorful Fruits and Veggies

Antioxidants are like the **bodyguards** of your **immune system**. They **protect your cells** from **damage, reduce inflammation**, and **support your health**. Here are some **foods** that are **rich in antioxidants**:

- **Colorful Fruits**: Fruits like **berries, cherries,** and **pomegranates** are **packed with antioxidants.** They **support your immune system** and **keep you healthy.**

- **Leafy Greens**: Leafy greens like **spinach, kale,** and **collard greens** are **rich in antioxidants** and **other nutrients** that **boost your immunity.**

- **Nuts and Seeds**: Nuts and seeds like **almonds, walnuts,** and **chia seeds** are **loaded with antioxidants** and **healthy fats** that **support your immune system.**

Malware Removal: Fighting Infection

Just like your computer needs **malware removal** to **keep it running smoothly**, your body needs **ways to fight infection** and **keep you healthy**. So, let's talk about **fighting infection** and **boosting your immune system**.

The Natural Remedies: Herbs and Spices

Herbs and **spices** are like the **natural remedies** that **boost your immune system** and **fight infection**. They **support your health** and **keep you protected**. So, let's talk about the **best herbs** and **spices** for **boosting your immunity**.

The Turmeric Tonic: Anti-Inflammatory Power

Turmeric is like the **super spice** that **boosts your immune system** and **fights inflammation**. It **contains curcumin**, a **powerful anti-inflammatory compound** that **supports your health**. Here are some **ways** to **incorporate turmeric** into your **diet**:

- **Turmeric Tea**: Brew a **soothing cup** of **turmeric tea** to **boost your immunity** and **reduce inflammation**.

- **Curry Powder**: Use **turmeric** in your **curry powder** to **add flavor** and **boost your health**.

- **Golden Milk**: Make a **warming cup** of **golden milk** with **turmeric, milk**, and **honey** to **support your immune system**.

The Garlic Guard: Antimicrobial Protection

Garlic is like the **natural antibiotic** that **fights infection** and boosts your immune system. It **contains allicin**, a **compound** that **kills bacteria** and **viruses**. Here are some **ways** to **incorporate garlic** into your **diet**:

- **Garlic Bread**: Make a **delicious loaf** of **garlic bread** to **boost your immunity** and **satisfy your taste buds**.

- **Stir-Fries**: Add **garlic** to your **stir-fries** for **extra flavor** and **immune support**.

- **Garlic Supplements**: Take **garlic supplements** to **boost your immune system** and **fight infection**.

The Probiotic Power: Gut Health

Probiotics are like the **good bacteria** that **support your gut health** and **boost your immune system**. They **help fight infection, reduce inflammation**, and **keep you healthy**. So, let's talk about the **best probiotics** for **boosting your immunity**.

The Fermented Friends: Yogurt and Kefir

Fermented foods like **yogurt** and **kefir** are **packed with probiotics** that **support your gut health** and **boost your immune system**. Here are some **tips** for **incorporating fermented foods** into your **diet**:

- **Yogurt**: Choose **plain, unsweetened yogurt** that **contains live cultures**. It **supports your gut health** and **boosts your immunity**.

- **Kefir**: Drink **kefir** for a **probiotic boost**. It **contains a variety** of **good bacteria** that **support your health**.

- **Sauerkraut**: Add **sauerkraut** to your **meals** for a **tangy, probiotic-rich** side dish.

The Supplement Solution: Probiotic Pills

Probiotic supplements are like the **convenient way** to **boost your gut health** and **support your immune system**. They provide a concentrated dose of **good bacteria** that **keep you healthy**. Here are some **tips** for **choosing probiotic supplements**:

- **Look for Live Cultures**: Choose supplements that **contain live cultures** to **ensure** you're **getting the most benefit**.

- **Check the Strains**: Look for supplements that **contain a variety** of **probiotic strains** to **support your gut health**.

- **Follow Instructions**: Follow the **recommended dosage** on the **label** to **ensure** you're **getting the right amount** of **probiotics**.

Security Updates: Strengthening Immunity

Just like your computer needs **regular security updates** to **keep it protected**, your body needs **ways to strengthen immunity** and **keep you healthy**. So, let's talk about **strengthening your immune system** and **boosting your health**.

The Exercise Effect: Boosting Immunity

Exercise is like the **system update** that **keeps your immune system** running smoothly. It **boosts your immunity, improves your health**, and **keeps you protected** from **illness**. So, let's talk about the **best exercises** for **boosting your immune system**.

The Cardio Kick: Aerobic Exercise

Aerobic exercise is like the **cardio boost** that **keeps your heart pumping** and your **immune system strong**. It **improves circulation, reduces inflammation**, and **supports your health**. Here are some **tips** for **incorporating aerobic exercise** into your **routine**:

- **Running**: Go for a **run** to **boost your immunity** and **improve your cardiovascular health**.

- **Cycling**: Hop on a **bike** for a **fun, immune-boosting workout**.

- **Swimming**: Take a **dip** in the **pool** for a **low-impact, immune-supporting exercise**.

The Strength Training: Building Muscle

Strength training is like the **muscle-building update** that **keeps your body strong** and your **immune system robust**. It **boosts your metabolism, improves your health**, and **supports your immunity**. Here are some **tips** for **incorporating strength training** into your **routine**:

- **Weightlifting**: Lift **weights** to **build muscle** and **boost your immune system**.

- **Bodyweight Exercises**: Use your **own body weight** for **effective, immune-supporting workouts**.

- **Resistance Bands**: Incorporate **resistance bands** into your **workouts** for a **challenging, immune-boosting routine**.

The Sleep Solution: Rest and Recovery

Sleep is like the **nightly reboot** that **keeps your immune system** running smoothly. It **repairs your body, reduces inflammation**, and **supports your health**. So, let's talk about the **importance of sleep** and **how to get the most** out of your **rest**.

The Sleep Stages: Understanding Your Rest

Your sleep is divided into **stages**, each with its own **unique benefits**. Understanding these **stages** can help you **optimize your sleep** and **maximize your immune support**.

- **Stage 1: Light Sleep**: This is
the **transition** from **wakefulness** to **sleep**. It's a **brief
stage** where your **body relaxes** and **prepares** for
deeper sleep.

- **Stage 2: Deeper Sleep**: During this stage, your **heart
rate slows, body temperature drops**, and your **body
prepares** for **deep sleep**.

- **Stage 3: Deep Sleep**: This is the **most restorative
stage** of sleep. Your **body repairs tissues, boosts your
immune system**, and **rejuvenates** your **brain**.

- **REM Sleep: Dream Time**: During REM (Rapid Eye
Movement) sleep, your **brain processes
information, consolidates memories**, and **prepares
you** for the day ahead.

The Sleep Hygiene: Tips for Better Sleep

Good sleep hygiene is like the **maintenance routine** that
keeps your immune system in **top shape**. Here are some **tips**
for **improving your sleep** and **boosting your immunity**:

- **Consistent Schedule**: Go to **bed** and **wake up** at
the **same time** every day, even on **weekends**.
This **consistency** helps **regulate your internal
clock** and **improve sleep quality**.

- **Create a Routine**: Establish a **bedtime
routine** that **signals** to your **body** it's time to **sleep**. This
could include **reading, taking a warm bath**,
or **listening to calming music**.

- **Optimize Your Environment**: Make your **sleep
environment** as **comfortable** and **conducive to
sleep** as possible. This includes a **cool
temperature, dark room**, and **comfortable bed**.

The Reboot: Starting Fresh

Alright, folks, it's time to talk about the **ultimate reset**—the **reboot** that **gets your system** back on track when things go **off the rails**. Think of it as the **factory reset** for your **biological supercomputer**. Sometimes, you just need to **hit the reset button** and **start fresh**. So, let's dive in and **hack into** the secrets of **rebooting your life**.

Factory Reset: When to Start Over

Just like your tech devices sometimes need a **factory reset** to **clear out the junk** and **get back to peak performance**, your life can benefit from a **reboot** every now and then. So, let's talk about **when to start over** and **how to know** when it's time for a **reset**.

The Red Flags: Signs You Need a Reboot

Red flags are like the **warning signs** that **tell you** it's time for a **reboot**. They **indicate** that something's **not right** and that you **need to make a change**. So, let's talk about the **common signs** that **signal** the need for a **reset**.

The Burnout Blues: Feeling Overwhelmed

Burnout is like the **system overload** that **leaves you feeling exhausted, overwhelmed**, and **ready to crash**. It's a **clear sign** that you **need a reboot** to **get back on track**. Here are some **symptoms** of **burnout**:

- **Chronic Fatigue**: Feeling **constantly tired**, even after **rest**. This is a **sign** that your **body** is **overworked** and **needs a break**.

- **Loss of Motivation**: Losing **interest** in things you **used to enjoy**. This can **indicate** that you're **overwhelmed** and **need to recharge**.

- **Increased Irritability**: Feeling **more irritable** or **short-tempered** than usual. This is a **sign** that your **body** is **under stress** and **needs a break**.

The Stagnation Station: Feeling Stuck

Stagnation is like the **system freeze** that **leaves you feeling stuck** and **unable to move forward**. It's a **sign** that you **need a reboot** to **get things flowing** again. Here are some **symptoms** of **stagnation**:

- **Lack of Progress**: Feeling like you're **not making any progress** in your **goals** or **aspirations**. This can **indicate** that you **need a fresh start**.

- **Boredom**: Feeling **bored** with your **routine** and **lacking excitement** in your **life**. This is a **sign** that you **need a change**.

- **Apathy**: Losing **interest** in things that **used to excite you**. This can **indicate** that you **need a reboot** to **reignite your passion**.

The Decision Point: Choosing to Reboot

Choosing to reboot is like the **decision point** where you **commit** to **making a change**. It's the **moment** when you **say**, "Enough is enough—it's time for a **fresh start**." So, let's talk about **making the decision** to **reboot** and **committing** to **change**.

The Pros and Cons: Weighing Your Options

Weighing your options is like the **cost-benefit analysis** that **helps you decide** whether a **reboot** is the **right choice** for you. Here are some **pros** and **cons** to **consider**:

- **Pros:**

- **Fresh Start**: A **reboot** gives you a **chance** to **start fresh** and **make positive changes**.

- **Improved Health**: Rebooting can **help you improve** your **physical** and **mental health**.

- **Increased Energy**: A **fresh start** can **boost your energy levels** and **help you feel more alive**.

- **Cons**:

  - **Disruption**: Rebooting can **disrupt** your **routine** and **require adjustments**.

  - **Uncertainty**: Starting over can **feel uncertain** and **scary**.

  - **Effort**: A **reboot** requires **effort** and **commitment** to m ake lasting changes.

The Commitment: Making a Plan

Making a plan is like the **blueprint** that **guides your reboot** and **helps you stay on track**. It **outlines** your **goals, strategies,** and **steps** to **achieve success**. Here are some **tips** for **creating a reboot plan**:

- **Set Goals**: Define your **goals** and **objectives** for your **reboot**. What do you **want to achieve**? What **changes** do you **want to make**?

- **Create a Timeline**: Establish a **timeline** for your **reboot**. When will you **start**? How long will it **take**? What are the **milestones** along the way?

- **Identify Resources**: Determine the **resources** you **need** to **support your reboot**. This could include **books, apps, support groups,** or **professional help**.

Safe Mode: Simplifying Your Life

Safe mode is like the **stripped-down version** of your **operating system** that **focuses** on the **essentials** and **eliminates distractions**. It's the **simplified approach** that **helps you reboot** and **get back to basics**. So, let's talk about **simplifying your life** and **focusing** on what **matters most**.

The Essentials: Focusing on What Matters

Focusing on the essentials is like the **core update** that **keeps your system** running smoothly and **eliminates unnecessary clutter**. It **helps you prioritize** what's **important** and **let go** of what's **not**. Here are some **tips** for **focusing on the essentials:**

- **Prioritize**: Make a **list** of your **priorities** and **focus** on what's **most important** to you. This **helps you stay focused** and **avoid distractions**.

- **Eliminate Clutter**: Get rid of **unnecessary clutter** in your **life**. This could include **physical clutter** like **junk** in your **home** or **mental clutter** like **negative thoughts**.

- **Simplify Routines**: Streamline your **daily routines** to **make them simpler** and **more efficient**. This **helps you save time** and **reduce stress**.

The Minimalist Mindset: Living with Less

Living with less is like the **minimalist update** that **keeps your system** lean and **efficient**. It **helps you focus** on what's **important** and **eliminate distractions**. So, let's talk about the **minimalist mindset** and **how to live with less**.

The Decluttering Process: Clearing Out the Junk

Decluttering is like the **system cleanup** that **removes unnecessary files** and **keeps your system** running smoothly. It **helps you eliminate distractions** and **focus** on what's **important**. Here are some **tips** for **decluttering**:

- **Start Small**: Begin with **small areas** of your **life** and **gradually expand**. This **makes the process less overwhelming**.

- **Be Ruthless**: Don't be **afraid** to **get rid of things** that **don't serve a purpose**. If it **doesn't add value, let it go**.

- **Organize**: Create a **system** for **organizing** your **belongings**. This **helps you stay clutter-free** and **keep things in order**.

The Simplicity Challenge: Embracing Minimalism

Embracing minimalism is like the **challenge** that **pushes you** to **live with less** and **focus** on what's **important**. It **helps you simplify your life** and **improve your well-being**. Here are some **tips** for **embracing minimalism**:

- **Set Limits**: Establish **limits** on how **many items** you **own** or **how much space** you **use**. This **helps you stay minimal** and **avoid clutter**.

- **Practice Gratitude**: Focus on **what you have** rather than **what you lack**. This **helps you appreciate** the **simplicity** of your **life**.

- **Seek Support:** Join **communities** or **groups** that **support minimalism**. This **helps you stay motivated** and **learn from others**.

System Restore: Revisiting Past Successes

System restore is like the **backup plan** that **helps you revert** to a **previous state** when things go **wrong**. It **allows you** to

revisit past successes and **learn from them** to **improve your future**. So, let's talk about **revisiting past successes** and **using them** to **guide your reboot**.

The Success Stories: Reflecting on Your Achievements

Reflecting on your achievements is like the **review** that **helps you understand** what **worked well** in the **past** and **how you can apply** those **lessons** to your **future**. Here are some **tips** for **reflecting on your successes**:

- **Make a List**: Write down your **past achievements** and **successes**. This **helps you see** what you've **accomplished** and **feel proud** of your **progress**.

- **Identify Patterns**: Look for **patterns** and **common themes** in your **successes**. What **strategies** did you **use**? What **lessons** did you **learn**?

- **Apply Lessons**: Use the **lessons** from your **past successes** to **guide your future**. What **worked well**? What **can you improve**?

The Learning Curve: Growing from Failure

Growing from failure is like the **learning curve** that **helps you improve** and **become stronger** after **setbacks**. It **teaches you** valuable **lessons** and **prepares you** for **future challenges**. So, let's talk about **learning from failure** and **using it** to **guide your reboot**.

The Failure Analysis: Understanding What Went Wrong

Understanding what went wrong is like the **debugging process** that **helps you identify** the **causes** of your **failures** and **learn from them**. Here are some **tips** for **analyzing your failures**:

- **Be Honest**: Be **honest** with yourself about **what went wrong**. What **mistakes** did you **make**? What **could you have done differently**?

- **Seek Feedback**: Ask for **feedback** from **others** who **witnessed your failure**. Their **perspective** can **provide valuable insights**.

- **Reflect**: Take **time** to **reflect** on your **failure**. What **lessons** did you **learn**? How **can you apply** those **lessons** to your **future**?

The Resilience Factor: Bouncing Back from Setbacks

Bouncing back from setbacks is like the **resilience** that **helps you recover** from **failures** and **keep moving forward**. It **strengthens your resolve** and **prepares you** for **future challenges**. Here are some **tips** for **building resilience**:

- **Stay Positive**: Maintain a **positive attitude** even in the **face of failure**. This **helps you stay motivated** and **keep moving forward**.

- **Set New Goals**: Use your **failure** as a **springboard** to **set new goals** and **challenges**. This **helps you stay focused** and **motivated**.

- **Seek Support**: Turn to **friends, family,** or **professionals** for **support** and **encouragement**. Their **help** can **make a big difference** in your **recovery**.

Epilogue: The Future of Human Debugging

Alright, folks, we've come a long way together. We've hacked into the mysteries of our biological supercomputers, debugged our systems, and optimized our operating systems. But the journey doesn't stop here. The future of human debugging is as exciting as it is unpredictable. So, let's take a peek into the crystal ball and see what lies ahead.

AI and You: Tech Innovations in Health

The future of health is all about **AI—artificial intelligence**. Imagine a world where **smart algorithms** can **predict** your **health issues** before they even happen. Where **wearable tech** can **monitor** your **vitals** in real-time and **alert** you to any **anomalies**. It's like having a **personal health assistant** that **never sleeps** and **always has your back**.

The Smart Health Assistant: AI in Action

AI-powered health assistants are like the **next-gen doctors** that **live in your pocket**. They **analyze** your **data, provide insights**, and **offer personalized recommendations**. Think of them as the **ultimate health coaches** that **know you better** than you **know yourself**.

The Data-Driven Diagnosis: Predictive Healthcare

Predictive healthcare is like the **crystal ball** that **foresees** your **health issues** before they **become serious**. It **uses AI** to **analyze** your **data** and **predict** potential **problems**. This **helps you take proactive steps** to **prevent illness** and **stay healthy**.

The Wearable Revolution: Real-Time Monitoring

Wearable tech is like the **fitness trackers** on **steroids**. They **monitor** your **vitals** in **real-time, track** your **activity levels**, and **provide insights** into your **health**. Imagine a **smartwatch** that **detects** a **heart issue** and **alerts** you to **seek medical attention**. It's like having a **personal doctor** on your **wrist**.

Next-Gen Upgrades: The Future of Longevity

The future of longevity is all about **next-gen upgrades—innovations** that **push the boundaries** of what's **possible**. Think **gene editing, nanobots,** and **personalized medicine**. It's like **upgrading** your **biological hardware** to **run faster, smoother,** and **longer**.

The Gene Editing Revolution: CRISPR and Beyond

Gene editing is like the **ultimate software update** for your **DNA**. It **allows scientists** to **modify** your **genes** to **correct defects, prevent diseases,** and **enhance your health**. Think of it as the **ultimate hack** that **rewrites** your **genetic code** for **optimal performance**.

The CRISPR Craze: Precision Gene Editing

CRISPR is like the **cutting-edge tool** that **makes gene editing** possible. It **allows scientists** to **precisely edit** your **DNA**, **correcting defects** and **enhancing your health**. Imagine a **world** where **genetic diseases** are a **thing of the past**. It's like **upgrading** your **genetic software** to **run flawlessly**.

The Ethical Dilemma: The Dark Side of Gene Editing

But with **great power** comes **great responsibility. Gene editing** raises **ethical questions** about **who** should **have access** to this **technology** and **how** it should **be used**. It's like the **double-edged sword** that **can cut both ways**. We **need to tread carefully** and **ensure** that **gene editing** is **used responsibly** and **ethically**.

The Nanobot Army: Microscopic Health Guardians

Nanobots are like the **microscopic soldiers** that **patrol** your **body, detecting** and **eliminating threats**. They **can deliver drugs, repair tissue**, and **monitor your health** in **real-time**. It's like having a **tiny army** of **health guardians** inside you.

The Drug Delivery System: Precision Medicine

Nanobots can **deliver drugs** directly to **targeted areas** of your **body, ensuring** that **medication** is **used efficiently** and **effectively**. Imagine a **world** where **cancer treatments** are **precise** and **minimally invasive**. It's like **upgrading** your **medical software** to **run smoother** and **more efficiently**.

The Tissue Repair Crew: Regenerative Medicine

Nanobots can also **repair tissue** and **promote healing**. They **can stimulate** the **growth** of **new cells** and **tissues, helping** your **body** to **regenerate** and **heal faster**. Imagine a **world** where **injuries** and **diseases** are **quickly repaired** and **healed**. It's like **upgrading** your **biological hardware** to **run faster** and **more efficiently**.

Staying Plugged In: Keeping Up with Health Trends

The future of health is **constantly evolving**, and **staying plugged in** is **crucial** for **keeping up** with the **latest trends** and **innovations**. It's like **updating** your **software** to **ensure** you're **running the latest version**. So, let's talk about **staying informed** and **keeping up** with the **future of health**.

The Health News Feed: Staying Informed

Staying informed is like **subscribing** to the **health news feed** that **keeps you updated** on the **latest trends** and **innovations**. It **helps you stay ahead** of the **curve** and **make informed decisions** about your **health**.

The Reliable Sources: Trusted Health Information

Trusted health information is like the **gold standard** for staying informed. It **comes from reliable sources** like **scientific journals, medical experts**, and **reputable organizations**. It **helps you separate fact** from **fiction** and **make informed decisions.**

The Social Media Buzz: Health Trends on the Rise

Social media is like the **buzzing hive** of **health trends** and **innovations**. It **keeps you connected** to the **latest news** and **trends** in the **health world**. But **beware** of the **misinformation** and **fake news**. Always **verify** your **sources** and **fact-check** your **information**.

The Health Community: Connecting with Like-Minded People

Connecting with like-minded people is like **joining** the **health community** that **supports** and **inspires** you. It **helps you stay motivated, learn from others**, and **share your experiences.**

The Online Forums: Sharing Knowledge and Support

Online forums are like the **virtual meeting places** where **people** come **together** to **share knowledge, support each other**, and **learn from one another**. They **provide a platform** for **discussion, advice**, and **encouragement.**

The Local Groups: Building Real-Life Connections

Local groups are like the **real-life communities** where **people** come **together** to **support** and **inspire each other**. They **provide opportunities** for **face-to-face interactions, shared experiences**, and **mutual support.**

Appendix: Cheat Codes & Easter Eggs

Alright, folks, we've covered a lot of ground in this guide, but no good hacker's manual would be complete without a few **cheat codes** and **Easter eggs**. Think of these as the **hidden gems** and **quick tips** that can **supercharge** your **health journey** and make life a little **easier** and **more fun**. So, let's dive in and **unlock** some **secret weapons** for your **biological debugging**.

Cheat Codes: Quick Tips for Success

Cheat codes are like the **shortcuts** and **tricks** that **help you achieve** your **goals** faster and **more efficiently**. They're the **hacks** that **save you time**, **effort**, and **frustration**. So, let's talk about some **quick tips** for **success**.

The Hydration Hack: Staying Hydrated

Staying hydrated is like the **ultimate cheat code** for **boosting your health** and **energy levels**. It **keeps your body** running smoothly and **supports all your systems**. Here are some **tips** for **staying hydrated:**

- **Drink Water Regularly**: Aim for **8 glasses** of **water** a day to **keep your body** well-hydrated.

- **Eat Hydrating Foods**: Foods like **fruits** and **vegetables** are **high in water content** and **can help keep you hydrated**.

- **Avoid Dehydrating Drinks**: Limit your **intake** of **caffeine** and **alcohol**, as they **can** dehydrate you.

The Sleep Solution: Better Rest

Better sleep is like the **cheat code** that **boosts your energy**, **improves your mood**, and **supports your health**. It **helps you**

wake up feeling **refreshed** and **ready to take on the day**. Here are some **tips** for **better sleep**:

- **Consistent Schedule**: Go to **bed** and **wake up** at the **same time** every day, even on **weekends**. This **consistency** helps **regulate your internal clock** and **improve sleep quality**.

- **Create a Routine**: Establish a **bedtime routine** that **signals** to your **body** it's time to **sleep**. This could include **reading, taking a warm bath**, or **listening to calming music**.

- **Optimize Your Environment**: Make your **sleep environment** as **comfortable** and **conducive to sleep** as possible. This includes a **cool temperature, dark room**, and **comfortable bed**.

The Exercise Boost: Quick Workouts

Quick workouts are like the **cheat codes** that **help you stay fit** and **healthy** without **spending hours** at the **gym**. They **provide a quick, effective way** to **boost your energy** and **improve your health**. Here are some **tips** for **quick workouts**:

- **High-Intensity Interval Training (HIIT)**: HIIT workouts are **short, intense bursts** of **exercise** followed by **brief rest periods**. They **burn calories** and **boost metabolism** in **minimal time**.

- **Bodyweight Exercises**: Use your **own body weight** for **effective, quick workouts**. Exercises like **push-ups, squats**, and **lunges** can be done **anywhere** and **require no equipment**.

- **Quick Cardio**: Go for a **quick run, bike ride**, or **jump rope session** to **get your heart pumping** and **boost your energy**.

Easter Eggs: Fun Health Hacks

Easter eggs are like the **hidden surprises** and **fun hacks** that **make your health journey** more **enjoyable** and **exciting**. They're the **little secrets** that **add a touch of magic** to your **routine**. So, let's talk about some **fun health hacks**.

The Laughter Cure: Boosting Mood and Health

Laughter is like the **ultimate Easter egg** that **boosts your mood, reduces stress**, and **improves your health**. It **releases endorphins**, the **feel-good hormones** that **make you happy** and **relaxed**. Here are some **tips** for **incorporating laughter** into your **life**:

- **Watch Comedy**: Enjoy **comedies, sitcoms**, and **funny movies** to **get your laugh on**.

- **Hang Out with Funny Friends**: Spend time with **people** who **make you laugh** and **bring joy** to your **life**.

- **Try Laughter Yoga**: Join a **laughter yoga class** to **experience** the **benefits** of **laughter** in a **group setting**.

The Nature Fix: Connecting with the Outdoors

Connecting with nature is like the **Easter egg** that **boosts your well-being, reduces stress**, and **improves your health**. It **helps you feel** more **grounded** and **connected** to the **world around you**. Here are some **tips** for **connecting with nature:**

- **Go for a Walk**: Take a **walk** in a **park, forest**, or **beach** to **enjoy** the **beauty** of **nature**.

- **Garden**: Start a **garden** and **spend time** tending to **plants**. This **helps you connect** with **nature** and **improve your well-being**.

- **Meditate Outdoors**: Practice **meditation** in a **natural setting** to **enhance** your **connection** with **nature** and **boost your well-being**.

The Music Therapy: Healing Through Sound

Music is like the **Easter egg** that **heals, soothes,** and **boosts your mood**. It **has the power** to **reduce stress, improve focus,** and **enhance your well-being**. Here are some **tips** for **using music** as **therapy**:

- **Create Playlists**: Make **playlists** for **different moods** and **activities**. Use **upbeat music** for **exercise** and **calming music** for **relaxation**.

- **Listen to Nature Sounds**: Enjoy the **sounds** of **nature**, like **birdsong, waves,** or **rain**, to **reduce stress** and **boost your well-being**.

- **Sing or Play an Instrument**: Engage in **musical activities** like **singing** or **playing an instrument** to **express yourself** and **boost your mood**.

www.ingramcontent.com/pod-product-compliance
Lightning Source LLC
Chambersburg PA
CBHW031328250726
48656CB00005B/2016